I0419463

Disclaimer:

The information contained herein is intended for educational purposes only. It is not the intent or purpose of the author or book to prescribe, diagnose, or treat specific ailments or prescribe special diets to those suffering with illness or disease. It is recommended that the health-seeker consult her/his health-care professional or doctor before making any radical changes in diet or lifestyle. The author assumes no responsibility for any changes brought about from following the information contained herein.

The Author

Plant-Based Nutrition: *A Human Perspective!*

Scope:

In an effort to evaluate the biological value of plant-based nutrition and its positive effectiveness of human wellness we take a critical look at the human body itself as clues to the direction of dietary intake. We also take a brief look into the "non-dietary" essentials of life in which neglect of their observance by the health-seeker means low-level health.

Rapid advances in the biological sciences as well as the creation of scientific tools which peer inside the inner resources of the human cell continue to give credence to the value of plant-based nutrition on human health and wellness. As we seek to ascertain the most appropriate and optimal food(s) for consumption in human nutrition important questions begin to emerge as to why particular foods are better fit to consume than others.

What evidence leads to the conclusion that plant foods are superior to animal foods, raw foods are superior to cooked foods, what makes onions and garlic poisonous to the body, why should fruits be eaten on an empty stomach, how can our emotions completely prohibit or aid in the digestion of the foods we eat, etc.

We then move on to highlight the fraudulent practices and dangerous assertions of the supplementation and pill-peddlers which permeate the world of dietetics. We then take a glimpse into what happens to the human body when food is withheld from it for a definite period of time and the physiological changes which occur as a result of abstinence from food.

Our discussion continues with the realization that human wellness is dictated and governed by physical and chemical laws. Likewise, digestion, absorption, and elimination of foodstuffs proceed in a unilateral direction in health and wellness and in the opposite direction under conditions of ill health. Humans are not exempt from following the laws of nutrition.

The amazing resilience of the human body is due in part to the immense innate wisdom endowed to it before birth.

Table of Contents

Chapter & Outline

Disclaimer

Scope

Forward
Joanne Russo

Credo of a Life Scientist
-T.C. Fry

Chapter 1
Structure Determines Function: *A Human Perspective!*

- I. Appraising the validity of plant-based nutrition through the structure of the human body.
  1. The blunt structure of the human teeth points to the dietary direction of plant foods over animal foods.
  2. Digestive secretions along the length of the gastrointestinal tract helps determine the efficiency in which foods eaten are properly digested and absorbed.
  3. The mind and the emotions are critical determining triggers to the overall fitness of the body to handle various foodstuffs properly and efficiently.

Supplementary Text Material: *The Great Power within You*
T.C. Fry

Chapter 2
Understanding our Dietary Place in the World

- II. Evaluating the overall "scheme" of humans on the "dietary tree" to determine dietary need.
  1. Anatomy, physiology, psychology, and the biological sciences give credence to the perspective that plant foods are superior to animal foods in human nutrition.

Chapter 3

Road to Superior Health: *Fasting Can Save Your Life*
- III. The human body prepares itself in times of special need.
  1. Fasting is defined as the withholding of food and drink (except water) until the return of hunger.
  2. Fasting continues as long as the food reserves of the body are sufficient to meet the needs of the body sustenance.
  3. Starvation is the withholding of food after the food reserves are exhausted and unable to sustain life.
  4. Breaking the fast properly is critical to the continued benefits of the fast.

Supplementary Text Material: *The Kidney: Master Organ of Waste Removal, Water Balance & Salt Balance*

Chapter 4
TrickTrition: *Lies, Lies, & More Lies...*
- IV. A critical discussion of manipulation & deception in the world of human nutrition.
  1. Disease and sickness has led to an exploitive industry directed towards health-seekers.
  2. The supplementation business is engaged in the largest human experiment in the world of dietetics. The results of which are increasingly disastrous.
  3. Pseudo-foods are becoming the norm and are replacing foods dictated by nature for human consumption.

Chapter 5
Superior Nutrition: *Life Subject to Law*
- V. Human nutrition is governed under strict biological law.
  1. Eating in accordance with physiological disposition means high-level health.
  2. Illness manifests itself after months or even years of dietary indiscretions.

Supplementary Text Material: *Questions from Health-Seekers*

Forward

Today there is much confusion and wrong advice concerning right consumption of food, i.e. fuel for our bodies.

There are many different ideas about what we are to eat for optimal health. Here in Health Truth Curtis Roberson gives clarity about what to eat, why the foods he proposes work best and the consequences of wrong eating which leads to the myriad of diseases we are encountering at a staggering rate today.

Here at last is the ultimate truth and we can know this is the truth because the foods listed here are in cooperation with the human body as it was meant to operate most efficiently, most optimally.

Back to the basics, back to the earth and the ground, to roots and plants, seeds and nuts, whole foods meant to be chewed and digested the old fashioned way. Here there are no pre-packaged or "other worldly" foods but only the whole apple closely picked to one's home state. Here we have the proper guidelines for where digestion begins, how it works before we even take a bite, how and why fasting is so vitally important for self-healing and why raw foods eaten in their natural state provide the most essential nutrients for our bodies, for our minds, for our souls.

My own journey into right eating, good health and nutrition began in 1981 as I couldn't eat the meat in college. When returning home to a home-cooked meal of meat I immediately became ill. The knowledge that stays in your colon for 4-5 days leaving a residue of toxins that could lead to colon cancer was also enough to propel me toward a plant-based diet. I came to realize our bodies house the Real Self, our Divine nature. As we honor and cherish ourselves we will naturally take care of the physical body which is the jacket for the spiritual body. I also began to read everything I could find on what makes for optimal health. My diet consisted mainly of macrobiotics, grains, beans and vegetables, as I naturally removed red meats, chicken and turkey, then fish from my diet. My diet evolved into almost no animal foods to what it is today, mostly raw, fresh and locally grown foods in season.

A raw vegan diet allows for inner tranquility, higher energy, and an intrinsic knowing we are eating fruits and plant vegetation from the earth we care about and wish to see thrive. Another reason I choose to be meat free is the idea the amount of grain needed to feed animals for growth can be used to feed humans; we can virtually end starvation in our world by the elimination of animal products.

According to PETA, People for the Ethical Treatment of Animals, *"we funnel huge amounts of grain, soybeans, and corn through all the animals we use for food instead of feeding starving humans. If we stopped intensively breeding farmed animals and grew crops to feed humans instead, we could easily feed everyone on the planet with healthy and affordable vegetarian foods."*

I have been a vegetarian for over two decades, going slowly toward a raw vegan diet. The way to incorporate change is to do it gradually, slowly eliminating animal foods, dairy products and foods that interfere with our optimal health.

In Health Truth we learn how eating food, not only which foods are best, but the importance of knowing when to eat and when to withhold, to fast from food when the body is in a state of ill health.

You will learn much from Health Truth, from Curtis Roberson's own personal journey and beliefs about right eating as he has over two decades of living a life in true health!

May your journey begin in light and love!

Joanne Russo, E-RYT

CREDO OF A LIFE SCIENTIST

I believe that life should be meaningful and filled with beauty, happiness and goodness.

I believe that humans are inherently good, righteous and virtuous, and I believe that their exalted character will be realized under ideal life conditions.

I believe that superlative well-being is normal to human existence and necessary to the realization of the highest human ideals.

Accordingly, to beget supreme human excellence, I embrace those precepts and practices productive of ideal life conditions for all.

I hold that **LIFE SCIENCE**, which encompasses all that bears upon human welfare, constitutes the only way to realize the highest possible order of human existence.

Therefore, I adopt **LIFE SCIENCE** as my way of life in the firm conviction that it and it alone, is in harmony with nature, in accord with the principles of vital organic existence, correct in science, sound in philosophy and ethics, in agreement with common sense, successful in practice and a blessing to humanity.

LIFE SCIENCE recognizes that the human body is a fully self-sufficient organism, that it is self-directing, self-constructing, self-preserving and self-healing, and that it is capable of maintaining itself in superb functioning order, *completely free of disease,* if its needs are met. Foremost among these are fresh air, pure water, rest and sleep, wholesome foods, cleanliness, comfortable temperature, sunshine, exercise, constructive work, emotional poise, self-mastery, recreation and pleasant environment.

LIFE SCIENCE recognizes that humans are constitutionally adapted to a diet of fruits, vegetables, nuts and seeds eaten in compatible combinations while in the fresh raw natural state.

LIFE SCIENCE recognizes that diseases are caused by improper life practices, especially dietary indiscretions. Illness proceeds from reduced nerve energy and consequent toxemia. Insufficient nerve energy arises from dissipation, stress, overindulgence, excess or deficiency of the normal essentials of life, or pollution of the body with substances not normal to it. Accordingly, recovery from sickness can be achieved only by discontinuing its causes and supplying conditions favorable to healing.

LIFE SCIENCE recognizes that a thoroughgoing rest, which includes fasting, is the most favorable condition under which an ailing body can purify and repair itself.

LIFE SCIENCE which teaches that exalted well-being can be attained and maintained only through biologically correct living practices, is not in any sense a healing art or a curing cult. It regards as mistaken and productive of untold grief the idea that diseases can be prevented or overcome by agencies abnormal to the body. Consequently, **LIFE SCIENCE** emphatically rejects all drugs, medications, vaccinations and treatments, because they undermine health by interfering with or destroying vital bodily processes and tissues.

Therefore, I regard my body as the inviolable sanctuary of my being. I insist that it is my inalienable right to have a pure and uncontaminated body, to be free of abnormal compulsions and restraints, and to be free to meet my needs as a responsible member of society

-T.C. Fry

Health Truth

Let us begin our journey into human wellness with an important concept which seems to elude writers of nutritional science. *'Health Truth'* is a unique term I am using here to describe the pursuit of accurate information in the employment of ascertaining and/or maintaining high-level health. But what exactly is truth? An internet search explains, *Truth* is a comprehensive term that in all of its nuances implies accuracy and honesty: *"We seek the truth, and endure the consequences" (Charles Seymour).* What is *'Health?'* Health is the absence of human biological degeneration. How can we evaluate the health status of health-seekers? How do we know if a person is healthy or not? How do we know what foods are sufficient to meet the biological and nutritive needs of humans? How do we determine what foods are positively harmful and contribute to degeneration? What are the 'non-nutritive' needs of human wellness? Pursuit of truth and understanding begins with pertinent questions that relates to the subject matter under discussion. For example, if the human body cannot or will not assimilate (digest and absorb) food under tremendous stress or in states of illness, does it not make sense to withhold food until the powers of assimilation and digestion are restored?

The ability to analyze and evaluate effective solutions to critical biological questions in the quest for health truth is of paramount importance in the application of scientific principles to human nutrition. I bid you to honestly consider an approach to wellness and longevity that is scientifically and biologically sound in principle and in practice.

"LET US HAVE THE TRUTH THOUGH THE HEAVENS FALL!"

The Beginning

My interest and fascination of the human body and how it functions began at the age of fourteen. Prior to this time I lived in a very dysfunctional home under the auspices of an uneducated mother. During the late 80's and the entire 90's my mother fell victim to the deadly crack cocaine epidemic. My father spent most of my childhood in and out of the penitentiary for various crimes, most notably the sale of crack cocaine. During this time there were a total of three siblings in the household myself included. There was no employment income in the household. My mother and father had little formal education; lacked motivation needed to succeed and, therefore relied on the welfare system as a means of providing food and shelter for the family. My mother's drug addiction skyrocketed out of control and she began to sell her welfare food stamps to feed her drug addiction. Once the food stamps were gone it left the family (myself and my year younger brother Antonio) scrambling to sustain ourselves from hunger for the rest of the month. To compensate my mother "created" meals out of flour, sugar, and other processed "foods" to sustain us for the rest of the month until the next date of the monthly food stamp allotment. This vicious cycle created a life of panhandling, especially for my brother Antonio which eventually led him through the gates of prison. Around the age of twelve my health began to deteriorate. I began having horrible headaches which eventually led me to having seizures. Having headaches were an everyday affair for me. At the age of nine I was prescribed high-blood pressure and seizure medication. I was placed in the care of family relative with my youngest brother Robert who was born with a developmental disability probably due to maternal drug abuse. Eventually my brother Antonio and I were placed into the foster care system at the tender ages of thirteen and fourteen. My seizures seemed to have discontinued by this time but the headaches I were having persisted. Then one day I picked up a book that began my transformation and renaissance into wellness and longevity. I learned that it is abnormal to be sick. I learned that not only was I living in a very toxic environment but, the foods I was eating contributed greatly to my deteriorating health condition. I made a "radical" decision to not only make a complete renovation of my eating habits but to pursue an unbiased scientific understanding of human wellness and transmit this information to as many health-seekers as I possibly could. To my amazement I no longer suffered with the long-standing headaches I suffered so long with. My seizures also subsided. I was able to completely discard the high-blood pressure and seizure medications I was taking at that time. During this time I also began my "academic" pursuit of scientifically understanding which foods were in consonance with body disposition and identifying those particular foods that contributed to ill health. Incorporating dietary changes to improve the quality of one's state of health is like climbing a muddy mountain in a rainstorm. I made a critical dietary change from an all processed animal-based diet to an all raw plant-based diet. My excitement was so complete for my new found health free from pain that I **NEVER** looked back. Over the years I decided to engage myself into nutritional and medical research and found myself scratching my head wondering why this information is not widely publicized and promoted by the medical profession and so-called nutritionists and dieticians as a means to maintaining and/or regaining high-level health. Then I finally realized that there isn't money in promoting **HEALTH TRUTH** to the general public. Just look around you and what do you see?

- **CHRONIC OBESITY**
- **POOR EYESIGHT**
- **HEART DISEASE**
- **ROTTEN TEETH**
- **CHRONIC FATIGUE**
- **ARTHRITIS OF VARIOUS MANIFESTATIONS**

- **DIABETES**
- **HYPERTENSION**
- **CANCER**
- **HEADACHES**
- **KIDNEY DISEASE**
- **GASTROINTESTINAL DISTURBANCES**
- **DISORDERS OF THE INTEGUMENTARY SYSTEM (SKIN)**
- **DISORDERS OF THE PANCREAS**
- **DISORDERS OF THE LIVER**
- **DISORDERS OF THE GALLBLADDER**
- **MUSCULAR DYSFUNCTION AND ABNORMALITIES**
- **BLOOD DISORDERS OF VARIOUS CELL TYPES**
- **ALTERATIONS IN MOOD AND EMOTION**
- **ANXIOUSNESS**
- **ANGER**
- **DEILITATING PAIN**

By no means is this list complete. This list highlights the sickness of humanity despite the arrogant boast of enlightened medicine that we are making extraordinary leaps and bounds of biological discovery to improve the quality of life of "modern-day" homo-sapiens.

Structure Determines Function

A Human Perspective

Chapter 1

CHAPTER OUTLINE

- **What does the structure and function of the human body tell us about the dietetic character of humans?**

- **How does body wisdom dwarf our conscious intellect?**

- **What is the 'concept of homeostasis' and how does it contribute to the overall wellness and survival of the human body?**

Most of the events that occur within the human body happen without any conscious involvement on the part of the organism. The human body is not a haphazard jumble of organs, skin, bones, and hair haphazardly mish-mashed together. There's an underlying intelligence that governs the internal complexity of the human body. There are literally millions of physiological[1] processes occurring simultaneously within the body without any conscious effort. So, what exactly does the position and structure of the organs and their secretions (or excretions) tell us about the nutritional needs of the human body at various stages of development? Look at the human teeth and their structure. The human teeth are very blunt and are not designed for "ripping and tearing" as so-called nutritionist and dieticians would have us believe. Humans like most other mammals develop two sets of teeth during a lifetime. The first of these teeth are called the *deciduous* or

---

[1] <u>Physiology</u>: is the scientific investigation into the function of the human body and its inner workings.

milk teeth, and they number 20 in humans. After the deciduous teeth are lost a permanent tooth replaces it and, there's additional 8-12 tooth appear bringing the total number of permanent teeth to 28-32 (including the four wisdom teeth). The human teeth are very blunt unlike the sharp teeth of canines. The human teeth are designed for crunching and grinding not tearing. The eyes of humans are situated practically in front of the face which is an indication that there is no need to be on alert to prepare the organism to chase down prey. Having a bipedal gait is another indication of humans' limited ability to chase down and apprehend food. What about the psychology of eating animals for food. It is quite repulsive to the psychology and emotions for humans to apprehend and rend a living animal for food consumption in the whole raw state. We can see just from the human anatomy that nature dictates the dietary disposition of humans. Let's now see what happens to animal and plant foods as they journey through the body. It is critical to get the most out of the food eaten. This means that the food eaten must be digested and absorbed if the body is to receive the nutrients it needs to conduct lifesaving activities such as healing wounds to maintain the integrity of the whole organism. This is accomplished via the **gastrointestinal system.** The human gastrointestinal system extends from the mouth to the anus. The adult gastrointestinal tract is a tube approximately 9 meters (30 feet) in length. That's right 30 feet! Can you imagine food rotting and decomposing in the body? Most of us are living with this toxic cesspool in our bodies. Exactly what foods decompose in this gastrointestinal system? That's right, **ALL ANIMAL PRODUCTS!** This decomposition builds over time, boils over into the blood, and leaves the victim suffering with debilitating chronic disease which eventually leads to cancer and premature death. Animal products are deficient in the nutrients needed to keep humans in a state of health and wellness. There are many control mechanism within the human body to prevent its early demise. This control mechanism is known as **'homeostasis.'**

What is homeostasis and how does it prevent damaging changes within the body? The basic living unit of the body is the cell. There are about 100 trillion cells in the human body. Each cell type whether it is lung, liver, skin, bone, kidney, or hair is specialized to perform a specific function to help maintain the integrity and survival of the organism. Although cells may differ markedly from one another there are certain basic characteristics they share in common. For instance, in all cells, oxygen is utilized to react with nutrients such as carbohydrates, fats, and proteins to liberate the energy required for the cell to perform its myriad functions. At the molecular, cellular and organ levels, structure determines function. Body cells must take in essential nutrients and eliminate wastes into its watery surroundings known as the "internal environment." Each of the 100 trillion cells of the body must participate in maintaining the appropriate composition of the internal environment in order to support the survival and functioning of **ALL** body cells. Therefore, homeostasis is the ability of the body to maintain a stable internal environment through various "check and balance(s)" which regulates and processes the integrity of its survival. Practically all physiological functions of the human body occur under the subconscious direction of the brain without any conscious awareness on the part of the organism. Innate intelligence and body wisdom exemplifies a higher consciousness at work when we witness the everyday poisoning of the human body with toxic food fare and outright rank poisons consumed on a daily basis as a normal way of life. Throughout this book we will call attention to these various poisons and provide a step by step program of self-assessment to release oneself from such dependency on these dangerous chemicals.

THE GREAT POWER WITHIN YOU
T.C. FRY

The following is an article written by health pioneer T.C. Fry based on the writings of the great Natural Hygienist, health educator and true Life Scientist, Dr. Herbert M. Shelton.

Living organisms are fully self-sufficient and self-governing entities. Supplied appropriately with the needs of life, they thrive in perfect health, completely free of disease. From conception all living organisms are endowed with a built-in program for a full, fruitful and joyous life. Living organisms are self-programmed to meet all life's needs within environments of their adaptation. All living organisms are self-directing, self-constructing, self-defending, self-preserving, self-maintaining, and, in the event of injury or illness, self-repairing or self-healing. *The healing principle is always in the living system itself.* The only power that can heal is the power that repairs; the only power that can repair is that power that produces; the power that now produces is the power that originally and always produced. *The power that constructs a full-grown individual from a fertilized ovum is the only healing power!*

Healing is, therefore, a continuous, unceasing and exclusively intrinsic power of every organism. The power that produces an organism and keeps it alive and functioning is the only power capable of governing, maintaining and healing it. Mastering and relying upon this great power within will yield a life of bliss and goodness *with complete freedom from ailments and suffering.* The simple, self-evident truth enunciated in this article embodies a long train of guiding principles that can enable you to avert miseries, woes and suffering. Knowing your tremendous inner capabilities frees you of many burdensome illusions and provides a key to true life enhancement. Recognizing the truth and implications of this message is the basis upon which you can immeasurably improve your life and its circumstances.

Recognizing the fundamental truth outlined in this message sets the stage for fulfilling the obligation you have to yourself and fellow beings, that of reorienting and reprogramming yourself for superlative well-being.

THE NEED FOR REPROGRAMMING YOURSELF

Standing in the way of total well-being for all too many who otherwise have the knowledge, the understanding and the dedication to achieve their highest potential are many ingrained bad habits, physiological addictions and erroneous concepts.

"Tis better to be ignorant than to know so much that isn't so."

Humans are creatures' habits. Habits are conditioned responses which we rely upon for personal efficiency. We spend many years from infanthood on learning responses to many thousands of situations and circumstances. With set response patterns we do not have to go through time-loss and trouble in solving problems anew every time we face them- we humans solve our problems once and for all and adopt the solutions as fixed and automatic responses known as habits. When situations reoccur, we unconsciously employ our habit patterns. That many of these habits amount to error fixation and that our accommodations to many of these habits amount to life-destroying perversions gives rise to the need to reprogram ourselves.

Most of our habits are learned from people who learned from others back into the murky reaches of time. Habits are always adapted and employed in accord with our own peculiar abilities.

Likewise, we learn most of our concepts and mis-concepts from others and adopt them in the shape or fashion our individual peculiarities dictate.

Habits are wonderful, for they are the foundation upon which our advanced human attainments have been built. As the most programmable beings in existence, we have more "conditioned responses" to carry us through more and greater complexities than other creatures in existence. By and large, our habits are constructive and get us along in this world remarkably well. On the hand, there are many "klunkers" in our armamentarium that sabotage our well-being.

Thus it follows that we can perform no better than the limitations of our self-programming. Our programming is at the same time our boon and our bane. To the extent that it guides us correctly, it is our boon. Insofar as it locks us into wrong conceptual frameworks, perverted outlooks, unwholesome practices, vitiated and antisocial dispositions and many other self-defeating characteristics, programming is a bar to our well-being.

It is unfortunate that most or all of us are incorrectly attuned to a greater or lesser extent in many of our life programs. But we are fortunate in that we, like computers, can be reprogrammed for better performance and more rewarding results.

If you want to capitalize upon the colossal potential within yourself, then you must reprogram yourself. Reprogramming yourself is difficult because you will be burdened heavily by the weight of previous conditioning and the drives, good, bad and indifferent, which initiate and impel your activities. You'll have to dispel a lot of myths and superstitions which infest your concepts and burden your thinking processes. What you take for granted is difficult to overcome. But you must and can do so.

To reprogram yourself for a better life on a higher plane of existence, the first order of business is to admit to yourself that you could harbor a lot of beliefs and practices that are responsible for you and your fellow beings' generally poor condition and overall suffering. We all know mental anguish and frustrations. These will flow from lives not led in accord with the course our innate nature decrees.

You can reprogram yourself to understand and practice the course you must follow. You can avoid those pitfalls that hamper you from assuming the position on the pedestal that all humans should occupy.

HOW TO REPROGRAM YOURSELF FOR SUPERLATIVE WELL-BEING

Following are the steps necessary for the ordinary person to become a Life Scientist, that is, to become an individual who conducts her or his life activities in accord with the dictates of the human biological heritage:

1. You must come to an awareness or knowledge that all is not right in this world of ours, or even with yourself. While almost everyone is self-satisfied that he or she has the answers to life's and society's vexations, the generally deteriorating condition of almost everyone seems to be self-evidence against such smugness. Therefore, you must be willing to admit to holding many erroneous notions. *We do not perceive our errors and often reject the truth when faced with it, but we must first, cultivate an open, receptive mind.*

2. You must seek knowledge and understanding with open arms. That you are reading this is in your favor. In seeking knowledge with the perspective of understanding, that is, wisdom, you'll be dependent upon your ability to master ideas and concepts.

3. You must seek knowledge, nonetheless, if you want to better your life situation. It is essential for correct reorientation. The fundamental principles, if applied on an individual and social scale, will salvage humanity from its depravity.

4. You must master an insight and understanding of what you learn-in your cosmogony you must fit all the parts and pieces of your knowledge such that you have perspective; it all must make good sense.

5. You must become the absolute master of your personal activities and circumstances. You must be willing, to the extent need dictates, to snap all ties with existing habits, intellectual stances and practices, no matter how deeply imbedded or how dear to you they may be.

6. You must be willing to end all fealty to anything that you *believe,* if need be. Keep in mind that the use of the word believe is a confession of ignorance, for it is not necessary to believe that which you know. To insist upon what you merely believe, may be insisting upon ignorance and misconception. Face up to the fact that many of your beliefs may be nothing more than myths and popularly-accepted superstitions that hamstring you.

7. You must be willing to change your circumstances, if necessary, to effect self-programming and to follow a correct life style.

8. You must undertake and study the conditions of health and well-being. Your greatest task is not the one of learning so much as unburdening yourself of a lot of burdensome intellectual baggage.

9. You must undertake to observe in your practices that which the truths you learn dictate.

This article lays the foundation of beginning change. Challenge yourself to incorporate new ideas and life practices on a continuing basis. Mastery of structure and function is an inherent biological adaptation which shows exquisite cooperation for survival of the human organism. The human body is not a jumble of skin, blood, bones, and hair jumbled together in a haphazard manner. Biological law is the underpinning of body function. The trillions of cells of the human body work symbiotically to maintain the highest functioning and survival of the whole body. Molecular, cellular, organ, and body structure and function pinpoints the true dietetic character of the human body. The coming chapters will provide further detailed evidence of the most optimal foods for total well-being. Concomitant to this evidence is information showing the "non-dietary" essentials of wellness. 'Health Excellence' is realized from living in accordance with biological law.

Understanding Our Dietary Place in the World!

Chapter 2

Let us begin our discussion with very pertinent questions in our quest to understand the true dietetic nature humans. If scientists have gathered sufficient information regarding how the body functions, why is there so much disagreement about the proper diet for humans? Is it true that humans who have practically the same anatomical and physiological features should follow different dietary practices? If an omnivorous (literally meaning an "everything eater") diet is the most appropriate dietary plan for humans then why are practically most of our ills diet-induced? Why should there ever be a need to eat processed foods?

America's dietary philosophy of eat and consume everything from grass to worms and everything in between has sent countless American's to an early grave and crippled countless more and, there seems to be no reprieve from such doom. Humanity's greed for dietary delicacy has created a ravenous destruction of plant and animal life to satisfy a perverted and depraved sense of taste. So-called *"enlightened"* humanity has toppled over every tree, lifted up every boulder and stone, dragged the bottoms of every large body of ocean, sea, and pond in a frenzied search for "esoteric nutrients" and the elixir of life. Complete consumption of an animal's muscle meat, eyes, bones, and fur has been an American dietary and cosmetic favorite for decades. Let's now turn our attention to some of the "favorite foods" we've come to enjoy and the harmful consequences which follow their ingestion.

Plant Foods vs. Animal Foods

-Cholesterol Content   -Water Content

-Vitamin Content   -Fiber Content

-Mineral Content   -Fulfillment of Enzyme Content

-Fat Content

To grasp and understand what particular foods are most optimal for human wellness and development, we must first understand the fact that the body needs nutrients for its survival to conduct very important life-saving physiological processes. Let's begin by stating the value of foods and their relative wholesomeness in human nutrition.

Criteria of Wholesome Foods:

- Level of Toxicity
- Edibility in the Uncooked (raw) state
- Taste Appeal (deliciousness)
- Ease/ Efficiency of Digestion
- Nutrient Adequacy (protein, vitamin, mineral salts, essential fatty acids, etc.)
- Fiber Content

- Water Content

- Fuel Value

- Sensory Appeal (are the senses in agreement of the look, feel, smell, etc., of the food?)

Animal Foods: In the human dietary animal foods and their by-products account for over 95% of the typical American diet. Consumption of animal foods and their by-products represent the greatest harm to human health and wellness. Animal foods and by-products of animal foods **DO NOT** meet one criteria of wholesomeness. Animal-based diets are continuing to kill American citizens despite "advances" in so-called medical science. Limiting animal foods in the diet is **NOT** enough. In "*FASTING and Eating for HEALTH* "*A Medical Doctor's Program for CONQUERING DISEASE*" Joel Furhman, M.D. quotes T. Colin Campbell, PhD explaining, "*There is strong evidence in the scientific literature that when a reduction in fat is compared to a reduction in protein intake, the protein effect on blood cholesterol is more significant than the effect of saturated fat. Animal protein is a hypercholesterolemic agent...Many Americans are switching from beef to skinless chicken and other animal-based foods simply to reduce their intake of fat. However the existing evidence suggests that this makes little or no sense.*"

Animal-based diets represent excessive protein and fat and increased premature death from chronic disease. Excessive animal protein in the diet means increased damage to the body. Increased loss of calcium in the urine occurs with the inevitable result of osteoporosis. Increased protein intake also means deterioration of kidney function. Excessive intake of animal foods especially meats of all kinds' means excessive ammonia and nitrogen generated through the metabolic process. **Ammonia intoxication** occurs because of elevated ammonia in the bloodstream. Symptoms may include tremors, slurred speech, vomiting, blurred vision, cerebral edema, and at high concentrations coma and death. Nitrogen enters the body in a variety of compounds present in food, most notably amino acids contained in dietary protein. **Nitrogen leaves** the body as **urea, ammonia,** and other products derived from amino acid metabolism. It critical to the health-seeker to understand that the human body is **NOT** equipped to handle animal foods and/or by-products of animal-based foods to any efficient degree without positive harm to the human body.

Joel Fuhrman, M.D. states, *"Urea is one irritating substance that results from excess protein. However, there are many other toxic by-products of protein metabolism besides urea that are not so easily measurable in the bloodstream. Researchers are finding that many of these other toxic by-products of protein digestion have a powerful toxic effect on the brain, and can cause mental fatigue and confusion as their levels rise in the body."*

Dr. Fuhrman continues, *"The liver is the major organ of detoxification and it is especially when the detoxification pathways in the liver are compromised that we see an increased likelihood that individuals will suffer from the toxic effects of their high-protein diets. A good way to illustrate the effect excess protein has on cerebral (brain) function is to look at patients with diseased livers. Patients with advanced stages of liver failure who cannot adequately metabolize excess dietary protein develop a change in mental function, drowsiness, confusion, and disorientation. They may eventually become markedly confused before lapsing into a coma. Dietary proteins, especially the ones containing sulfated amino acids and aromatic amino acids—from the proteins contained in animal products—must be significantly curtailed in patients with liver disease. This is the established treatment for this condition. Without restricting animal proteins, their mental condition will significantly worsen.*

A crucial point to keep in mind here is that there are 14 other toxins besides urea that are breakdown products of protein metabolism. Even though urea is the only one we can inexpensively measure in the bloodstream at this time, the other protein-related toxins are more responsible than urea for the mentally confused state we see in cirrhotic individuals.

Uric acid and other potentially harmful nitrogenous wastes such as ammonia increase in our body when we consume excessive protein. Vegetable proteins generate less ammonia and other harmful wastes and are less acid-forming as well."

This statement by Dr. Fuhrman illustrates the mandatory need to completely eliminate animal foods from the diet if we are to realize long-term well-being. More importantly, there is a major distinction between humans and wild animals that are true carnivores in which meat is the primary source of their nutritive diet. What is this major distinction? Animals that are primarily flesh-eating consume their meat in the raw state. This means that human primarily eat their meat with the assistance of **HEAT**. Cooked proteins produce toxic changes; distort the chemical composition of the protein molecule on the molecular level, and leaves *toxic* debris in the system that the body must dispose of. The protein molecule is so complex and large that they're known as *"macromolecule[2]s."* The individual amino acids that make up the protein molecule are destroyed and rendered useless as vital food factors to the extent they are destroyed by the cooking process. These destructive changes occur in all essential and "nonessential" amino acids. The length of the gastrointestinal tract dictates which foods are superior for human nutrition. The gastrointestinal tract is a *"living"* tube that is specialized along its length for the sequential processing of food. The alimentary canal is about 15ft. in length. This is quite considerable. It

---

[2] Macromolecule: A very large molecule formed by the joining of smaller molecules.

reasons that the health-seeker understands the proposition that foods the eaten should be the most easily digested, absorbed, and eliminated.

Let's now turn our attention to the intimate details of human digestion and how the body prepares itself the incoming array of vitamins, minerals, enzymes, fiber, water, and other vital substances so critical to its continued survival.

Biological Integrated Response to a Meal[3]

This discussion explores the biological, psychological, physical, and physiological mechanisms at play that ensure the efficient entrance, digestion, absorption, and utilization of nutrients from foodstuffs eaten.

'Brain-Gut Axis[4] of Human Digestion'

---

[3] The biological integrated response to a meal: reflects the control mechanisms at play to ensure proper processing, delivery, absorption, and elimination of foodstuffs within the human body.

[4] Brain-Gut Axis: refers to the interplay of communication between the brain and gastrointestinal system for optimal processing of the ingested meal.

Psychology of Digestion

Cephalic-Phase of Digestion: The cephalic-phase of digestion refers to the mind where thoughts are generated. In other words, thinking about food, the thought of food, or the utterance of food, especially when we are hungry send signals throughout the body for preparation of a meal. In this stage of preparation for a meal the gastrointestinal tube is called into *"action"* in readiness for the incoming meal. The primary stimuli at this stage of preliminary digestion is psychological in nature through the process of thinking about the consumption of food, olfactory and sensory input (the smell of appetizing food, or seeing food when hungry), and auditory input (hearing others speak about food).

Oral-Phase of Digestion: The oral-phase of digestion quickly follows the cephalic-phase. Both phases can be said to be interlinked because the cephalic-phase of digestion involves neural input to begin salivary secretion. The primary difference is that during the oral-phase of digestion food is in contact with the physical surface of the gastrointestinal tract. Additionally, the physical digestion of food begins in the oral cavity (mouth). Carbohydrate digestion begins in the mouth with the enzyme *salivary amylase.* Saliva plays a critical role in the facilitation and initiation of the digestion of food. Saliva lubricates and moistens food for ease of swallowing, initiates carbohydrate digestion, neutralizes refluxed acidic contents in the esophagus, and maintains the integrity of the oral cavity through antibacterial activity.

Esophageal-Phase of Digestion: The esophagus is a muscular tube about 10 inches long. The passage of food from the esophagus to the anus is controlled by muscles called *"sphincters"* strategically located to prevent backflow of digestive contents. Swallowing is initiated voluntarily, but once it has been initiated, it cannot be stopped. During the esophageal-phase of digestion the **swallowing center** located in the *medulla* (brain) initiates a **primary peristaltic wave** that sweeps from the beginning to the end of the esophagus, forcing the *bolus* (food that has been swallowed). No digestion or absorption of nutrients occurs in the esophagus. The entire transit time of food from the pharynx, esophagus and, stomach averages a mere 6-10 seconds. Additionally, during the esophageal-phase of digestion the secretion of the esophagus is entirely protective in nature. Mucus is secreted throughout the length of the gastrointestinal tract to provide lubrication for the passage of food to decrease the likelihood of the esophagus being damaged by any sharp edges in the newly incoming food. There's additional mucus protection of the esophageal wall from acid and digestive enzymes in gastric juice, if gastric reflux should unexpectedly happen.

Gastric-Phase of Digestion: During the next stage in the physiological response to a meal, food enters the stomach. Just below the esophagus, the gastrointestinal tract expands to form the **stomach**[5], which temporarily stores food and begins the digestion of protein. There are **3** primary functions of the stomach:

1. The stomach stores ingested food until it can be emptied into the small intestine at an appropriate pace for efficient digestion and absorption. It requires many hours to digest and absorb a meal that took only minutes to consume.

2. The stomach secretes hydrochloric acid (HCI) and various enzymes to begin the digestion of protein. There are numerous cells in the wall of the stomach to effectively and efficiently begin the digestion of protein. The anatomical features (muscle layers) of the

---

[5] The stomach serves 3 primary functions: (1) storage of large quantities of food until it can be processed; (2) mixing of the food with gastric secretions until it forms a semifluid mixture called *chyme;* (3) slow emptying of the chyme from the stomach into the small intestine at a rate suitable for proper digestion and absorption by the small intestine.

stomach allows it to not only mix, churn, and move food along the digestive tract, but also to pummel the ingested food, physically breaking it down into smaller fragments, and to push the food into the small intestine (which is where most absorption of nutrients occurs).

3. The mixing, pulverizing, and propulsive movements of the gastric contents are mixed with gastric secretions to produce a thick liquid mixture called *chyme* (a thick liquid mixture of food and digestive juices). Gastric contents must be converted to chyme before moving on into the duodenum (the first segment of the small intestine).

Intestinal-Phase of Digestion: The small intestine is where most absorption and/or assimilation of nutrients occur. The most critical aspect of the small intestinal phase in response to a meal is the controlled and precise delivery of chyme from the stomach into the small intestine. All of these physiological activities are exquisitely coordinated under the direction of the brain via neural input. Additionally, secretions from the pancreas and biliary system (liver, gallbladder, and associated ducts) are called upon in a coordinated fashion for optimal and efficient handling of intestinal contents for ensuring proper digestion and absorption. The **liver** is the largest and most critical metabolic organ in the human body. The can be viewed as the body's biochemical transformation factory. The liver performs a multitude of functions that are critical to the continued survival of the human body:

- The liver is the storage site for many critical nutrients such as vitamins and minerals.
- The liver stores iron.
- Fat metabolism; Carbohydrate metabolism; Protein metabolism.
- Detoxification and/or breakdown of body wastes and hormones, including drugs and foreign substances.

- Activation of vitamin D, which the liver accomplishes in conjunction with the kidneys.

- Removal of bacteria and worn-out red blood cells.

- The liver has the unique ability of self-renewal or regeneration from injury.

This short list shows just how important a role the liver plays in maintaining the integrity of the human body for continued survival.

__Colonic or Intestinal-Phase of Digestion__: The most distal (farthest away from the mouth) segment of the gastrointestinal tract is called the **large intestine**. The large intestine receives components of the meal that are indigestible (such as cellulose), reabsorb the remaining fluid that was used during movement of the meal along the digestive tract, and finally store the metabolic waste products of the meal until they can be appropriately eliminated from the body. The large intestine is primarily a drying and storage organ.

Unique to the large intestine is its biological ecosystem of intestinal flora (commensal bacteria) numbering in the trillions, providing a critical symbiotic relationship with the host by providing metabolic functions that are vital to intestinal health (such as metabolizing components of the meal not digested by host enzymes) and, making their products available to the body via a process known as **fermentation**. Evidence shows that the microbial environment of the colon is also capable of detoxifying drugs and other substances that threaten the integrity of the human body. The lining of the intestine is renewed at an extraordinary rate. Amazingly, the entire intestinal tract is renewed every 4-5 days. This event shows just how efficient and powerful the mechanisms within the human are body dedicated to optimal and efficient function. Scientific studies are describing a genetic hierarchy responsible for cell fate commitment (inherent commitment to the organisms' survival) in normal gut physiology.

This brief and limited survey of human physiology is intended to give the health-seeker a very basic perspective of the *"internal wisdom"* inherent within the human body. This vital information is intended likewise to spur intellectual curiosity and further exploration into the intimate details of psychological, anatomical, and physiological function and to synthesize this information into a true and logical basis of human wellness.

Nutritional Basis of Life

We will now turn our attention to the *"nutritional basis of life"* and give a comprehensive treatment of those chemical substances which are the very basis of keeping the body functioning on a daily basis.

Concept of homeostasis[6]

The human body contains about 100 trillion cells. When we contemplate the complexity and physiological diversity of the many function performed by the body we have to wonder why very little goes wrong with this remarkable organism. The body's ability to maintain internal stability and/or equilibrium of internal conditions such as bodily fluids, physiological cooperation of internal organs, and maintenance of a dynamic steady state of the internal environment is termed *homeostasis*. *Homeostasis is critical to the survival of each cell, and each cell, through its specialized cellular activities, contributes to the maintenance of the internal environment shared by all cells.*

HARMFUL PRATICES TO AVOID

---

[6] <u>Homeostasis:</u> is maintenance and stability of the internal environment of the body in which the cells live. It is absolutely critical to the continued survival of the body as a whole.
(*homeo* means "the same"; *stasis* means "to stand or stay").

The Case Against "Nutritional" Supplements

There is a preponderance of scientific evidence to support the fact that the present health status of the American people and, people around the globe is in a degenerate state. Scientists and health-care professionals in the medical community argue that the modern diet is deficient and requires nutritional supplementation with certain nutrients in order to bridge the gap of this deficiency. The inherent power within the body that has brought it from the embryonic stage of life to a full grown adult is the same biological mechanism that will maintain and keep the human body in a state of superior wellness when provided with foods mandated by biological disposition. Consumption of nutritional supplements is akin to going directly to the soil and eating it. Nature hands up nutrients that have been elaborated upon by the plant kingdom through the complex process of photosynthesis. There is a crucial symbiotic relationship which exists between and among the various nutrients. Nutrients **do not** have separate and isolated functions but are used as a harmonious interrelated team. When this *"nutritional bond"* is broken through fragmentation the biological effectiveness of the nutrient is severely handicapped. The idea of using supplements as a means to *"cure"* a diseased condition or provide increased biological energy is complete folly. Supplementation is an attempt to undermine organic law. For example, it is a well-known fact that chemical laws undergird life's biological processes. We cannot possibly undermine this inherent physiological mandate of human life. There is a very unique and complex nutrient synergism which exists between various metabolic and organ systems within human physiology. In doing so, we are bankrupting our pockets and compromising the quality of our well-being. Stuffing the body full of unusable toxic so-called *"nutritional supplements"* causes a serious toxic condition on one end and the potential for a serious disease condition on the other. It has been stated that the consumption of *"supplementary substances is* *the largest nutritional experiment in the long history of the human race, the results of which are not yet in nor ready for evaluation. The great increase in chronic degenerative catastrophic diseases would appear to negate the well-touted concept that using supplements is beneficial."* I can say with confident conviction that the evidence of supplementation being positively harmful is clear as with the rising sale of these poisons, with a concomitant rise of chronic degenerative disease among health-seekers. The principles of nutrition are not subject to change. *All humans are fundamentally alike with similar organs, systems and cells which may vary in efficiency of performance but not in their method of function.* The primary danger posed by nutritional supplementation is *overnutrition.* The human body is called upon to dispose of this excess, and in the process the kidneys and liver are severely overworked and energy reserves wasted and loss. Selling vitamins, minerals, enzymes, and other nutrient elements is a very profitable business, coming at the expense of the health-seekers well-being. Proprietors of supplements are now proclaiming that their products are *"organic"* and therefore acceptable. What about the nutrients that are *"undiscovered?"* There is a vast body of knowledge of biological phenomenon that is yet to be explored and scrutinized for the benefit of human wellness. The self-healing mechanisms of the human body allow pathology to continue unchecked while the health-seeker is deluded into a false since of well-being. Consider the statement, *"Vast realms of the human life motif are yet to be explored and resolved in finality. Millions of people taking vitamins are willing guinea pigs in a vast experiment, the results of which are, by the measure of things, completely unknown and unpredictable in the absence of long-term and precise evidence."* Anyone interested in *"nutritional superiority"* will follow the dictates of nature and consume those foods which are package by the hand of biological law and not *"put together"* by the finite, arrogant mind of fallible science.

The Case Against Herbs and Herbal Supplements

Herbs are defined as, *"any plants with leaves, seeds, or flowers used for flavoring, food, medicine, or perfume"* or parts of *"such a plant as used in cooking."*

Herbs have been used to treat the *"ills of the flesh"* since time immemorial. There are those who wish to divorce the herbal practice from the medical practice insisting on the notion that herbs are *"natural"* and that they originate from *natural* sources. *Natural* **does not** necessarily mean beneficial. These so-called beneficial properties the peddlers of herbs scream about are actually the toxic drug-effects witnessed after administration or consumption of the poisonous chemicals. It is critical for the health-seeker to understand that herbs are **"inert[7]"** and have no special or inherent abilities to impart wellness, longevity, or increased body energy in any way. It is precisely because of their *poisonous* effects on the human body that herbs are so effectively promoted. Consider the assertions for *"curing"* disease and/or disease condition(s) for herbs made by so-called herbalists:

- Enlarged prostate
- Common cold
- Headaches
- Allergies
- Cancer
- Eczema
- Muscle spasms
- Bruised spleen

---

[7] Inert: refers to absolute inactivity; lacking the ability or strength to move; having no ability to perform action.

- Heart disease

This list is by no means complete. There are literally hundreds of disease conditions herbs are said to *cure.* The fact that herbs are relied upon as substances that disrupt and alter body function is indicative of their inherent toxic qualities and **<u>cannot</u>** be relied upon as substances capable or appropriate for building blood, bone, flesh, and renewal of body tissue so critical for the body's continued survival. Herbs fail to meet a number of critical criteria[8] of wholesomeness mentioned earlier. One criterion is that food **must be nontoxic**. Of course, herbs fail to meet many of the biological criteria mandated by the human body as a source of nutritional value.

Road to Superior *Health:* FASTING CAN SAVE YOUR LIFE

Chapter 3

<u>CHAPTER OUTLINE</u>

- **Fasting is the quickest, safest, and most efficient method of internal bodily cleansing and healing employed (instinctually) in the living world.**
- **Employment of fasting allows physiological rest and increased elimination of the products of cellular metabolism.**

---

[8] <u>Criteria</u>: Are a set of principles or standards by which something may be judged or decided; a set of requirements deemed mandatory for acceptance.

- Fasting <u>does not</u> *cure* disease but allows the body more efficient control *(under the direction of the brain)* of physiological processes and calls into play internal mechanisms to purposefully handle and dispose of unwanted excess.

"Fasting enables the processes of renewal to outdistance the processes of degeneration and the result is a higher standard of health. Regeneration of the flesh, even the very marrow of the bones, is possible through this method. By fasting we may actually tear down much of the body and then rebuild it."

-Herbert M. Shelton

The public has been and continues to be gravely misinformed regarding accurate information needed to make critical decisions regarding their health and well-being. Practically *all* health-seekers are suffering from degenerate health. Medical *science* offers continued *"cures"* for disease conditions caused from living contrary to biological disposition.

Dr. Shelton states, *"The **Hygienic System** is not a system of treating and **curing** <u>diseases</u> and <u>disorder</u>. It does not recognize the existence of hundreds, or thousands of <u>diseases</u>, but regards all of these many so-called <u>diseases</u> as varying expressions of the same thing. **Hygienic** methods are methods of caring for the body. By these we seek to place the body under the most favorable conditions for the prosecution of its own healing activities."*

This statement exemplifies the fact that the human body is the primary master of its own internal domain. So, exactly what is fasting[9]?

Fasting is complete and voluntary elimination and withholding of <u>ALL</u> food with the exception of pure water until the return of hunger.

---

[9] <u>Fast</u>: is derived from the Anglo-Saxon word, *faest*, which means "firm" or "fixed." Fasting is voluntary and entire abstinence from all food except water.

There is instinctual repugnance to food when the organism is in a state of illness, seriously injured, or emotionally excited or disturbed. This aversion to food is nature's method of cutting off the appetite of the organism to allow for physiological processing.

Dr. Shelton describes how fasting allows the body to self-heal:

- **It gives the vital organs a complete rest.**
- **It stops the intake of foods that decompose in the intestines and further poison the food.**
- **It empties the digestive tract and disposes of putrefactive bacteria.**
- **It gives the organs of elimination an opportunity to catch up with their work and promotes elimination.**
- **It re-establishes normal physiological chemistry and normal secretions.**
- **It promotes the breaking down and absorption of exudates, effusions, deposits, "diseased" tissues, and abnormal growths.**
- **It restores a youthful condition to the cells and tissues and rejuvenates the body.**
- **It permits the conservation and re-canalization of energy.**
- **It increases the powers of digestion and assimilation.**
- **It clears and strengthens the mind.**
- **It improves function throughout the body.**

This short list gives a critical glimpse into the powerful efficiency of how the human body harnesses the internal resources of its nutritive reserves and dispose of excess toxic cellular debris. Let's now take a more in-depth journey into the actual fast from beginning to end.

How to Begin the Fast: Fasting should not be approached as a trying and difficult idea or concept. There are many and varied prejudices against the fast that needs mention here.

1. It is stated that *fasting* and *starvation* is synonymous, meaning they are one and the same.

2. It is stated that *fasting* injures vital organs such as the heart.

3. It is stated that *fasting* for any considerable length of time is positively dangerous.

While the body itself is the foremost *"authority"* regarding when to fast, the duration of the fast, and the appropriate time to resume eating, it is <u>critical</u> that the health-seeker approach fasting with caution if considering this method because of serious ill health to secure the expertise of a competent professional who is familiar with the contra-indications to fasting and who can accurately evaluate any and all symptomology of the fast.

The fast should be entered upon with great anticipation of change. Fear of abstinence from food is unfounded and typically based upon ignorance or misinformation regarding the internal resources of the human body to sustain itself when food is withheld for a definite period of time.

The brain exercises exquisite control over the nutritive needs of the human body. Fasting *begins* with the discontinuance of all food (except water) and is sustained and/or maintained while the nutritive reserves of the body are sufficiently adequate to support the physiological processes of the organism and *ends* when those reserves are *exhausted* and no longer capable to meet the demands of nutritional support, at which point *starvation* becomes imminent.

While researching fasting via the internet I came across an interesting link on fasting entitled, *"Health and Medical Articles:"* The Dangers of Fasting. The article states, *"...fasting has fewer advantages than disadvantages and most people don't know how dangerous fasting is."*

"It affects not only our physical being, but our mental, emotional, and spiritual self as well. But why and how it endangers our health whilst some scientists say it will do us good? Well, let's see... Because of the lack of glucose consumed, the liver converts glycogen stores into glucose and energy. The brain and the central nervous system need direct glucose, so they must

get it either from the breakdown of proteins, so fatty acids, after being converted into ketones, become the primary source of energy. **Ketosis**[10] is subdued by drinking plenty of fruit juices, which provide simple carbohydrates for energy and cellular functioning."

"Some diets restrict all solid foods and instruct dieters to survive on only low-calorie beverages for days at a time. The Joshi holistic diet involves an elaborate list of so-called acid-forming foods to avoid for three weeks, including seemingly healthy vegetables and cereals."

"If you decide to follow such a diet or to fast for detox your body or for any other reasons, you should think twice and consider the side-effects: headaches, nausea, and muscle aches. Everyone responds to detoxification differently, depending on the level of toxicity in the body. While one person's body becomes sick immediately after beginning a fast, another person may feel energized and renewed. These side effects include a drop in blood pressure, a persistent cold, and acute emotional distress. Still, depriving the body of the vitamins and minerals you get from food weak the body's ability to fight infections and inflammation."

"A prolonged fast/diet can lead to anemia, impairment of liver function, kidney stones, mineral imbalances, and other undesirable side effects. Deaths due to prolonged fasting have occurred, usually in people who believe this would "purify" their body or cure them of some disease. Moreover, for people with diabetes taking certain tablets and/or insulin to manage their condition, the dangers are much higher. If you are a diabetic and you are intending to fast, you should attend your diabetic clinic for an assessment of your current level of diabetes control because the greatest danger is that of hypoglycemia[11]. There is also the danger of the blood

---

[10] Ketosis: is the presence in the blood of certain end-products of fat metabolism, known as ketones. There are three ketones- acetoacetic acid, acetone, and beta-hydroxybutyric acid.
[11] Hypoglycemia: is characterized by low blood glucose.

glucose level becoming too high when normal levels of medications are not taken. This can lead to diabetic ketoacidosis (DKA[12]), a condition requiring hospital admission.

Therefore, you should pay attention to what you eat and how you eat and try to avoid fasting as much as you can. *Always remember that health is more important than silhouette, sicknesses have medical cures and you don't have to starve yourself to death for that. And if you are a religious person in search for divine communication or Nirvana, well... maybe your faith is stronger than your health."*

Let us expose this continued *echo of ignorance* against fasting by those who are grossly unqualified to speak about the efficaciousness or biological value of the fast. We will begin by tearing apart this rambling jumble of empty words and replace them with biological and physiological fact.

Let's see what the writer says and provide a counter-argument in favor of biological fasting:

1. **Statement**: The writer says, *"fasting has fewer advantages than disadvantages and most people don't know how dangerous fasting is."*

    Rebuttal: Fasting is dangerous in the minds of the uninformed and those lacking scientific know-how to interpret correctly the physiological processes occurring within the human body when food is withheld for an indefinite period of time.

2. **Statement**: The writer says (of fasting), *"It affects not only our physical being, but our mental, emotional, and spiritual self as well. But why and how it endangers our health whilst some scientists say it will do us good?*
    *Well, let's see...Because of the lack of glucose consumed, the liver converts glycogen stores into glucose and energy. The brain and central nervous system need direct glucose, so they must get it either from the breakdown of proteins, so fatty acids, after being converted into ketones, become the primary source of energy. **Ketosis** is subdued by drinking plenty of fruit juices, which provide simple carbohydrates for energy and cellular functioning."*

---

[12] Diabetic Ketoacidosis: results from shortage of insulin; inn response the body switches to *"burning"* fatty acids to meet its energy needs.

Rebuttal: The writer leaves us in the dark about how fasting affects our physical, mental, emotional, and spiritual self. I suspect it's because the writer is likewise clueless. The liver ONLY converts glycogen (which is the body's storage from of glucose) into glucose after the superfluous tissue such as fat has been efficiently utilized to meet the energy needs of various tissues in the body. The human body does not indiscriminately break down protein to meet the needs for energy. Structural proteins are practically "untouched" under the condition of fasting. We see an actual increased efficient use of amino acids and proteins after the fast. The brain will actually use ketones as an alternative fuel source to support the energy needs of other metabolic tissues in the body. The statement the writer makes about **ketosis** is utterly ridiculous. Ketones are a metabolic product of lipid or fat metabolism used by various cells as an alternative fuel source. When carbohydrates are insufficient to meet the needs of the body ketones are used as an emergency energy source particularly during fasting or starvation. This is biological wisdom at its best. The human body controls this critical survival mechanism. The writer gives no explanation as to why ketosis should be *subdued by drinking plenty of fruit juices, which provide simple carbohydrates for energy and cellular functioning."*

3. **Statement**: The writer says, *"A prolonged fast/diet can lead to anemia, impairment of liver function, kidney stones, mineral imbalances, and other undesirable side effects. Deaths due to prolonged fasting have occurred, usually in people who believe this would "purify" their body or cure them of some disease. Moreover, for people with diabetes taking certain tablets and/or insulin to manage their condition, the dangers are much higher.*

   Rebuttal: Fasting cannot possibly lead to anemia, impairment of liver function, kidney stones, mineral imbalances, or undesirable side effects. Fasting is a *cessation of doing.* Fasting allows the internal resources of the body to dictate increased elimination and removal of poisons and by-products of cellular metabolism from the body in a very efficient manner. To say that fasting may lead to anemia is beyond the height of absurdity. Anemia is a reduction or deficiency of hemoglobin, the oxygen-carrying protein of red blood cells. Dr. Herbert M. Shelton provided scientific certainty and very interesting case studies that fasting cannot and does not cause anemia even under the most prolonged fasting cases. The physiological value of fasting has been and continues to be demonstrated in the scientific community. The medical management of diabetes has sent countless diabetics to their deaths from treatment and grossly misguided and inappropriate dietetic advice. All animal foods (which are excessively high in saturated fat) has been shown to be the primary and major causative factor in development of diabetes and that treatment with insulin contributes to the acceleration of death from the diabetic condition.

4. **Statement**: The writer says, *"If you are a diabetic and you are intending to fast, you should attend your diabetic clinic for an assessment of your current level of diabetes control because the greatest danger is that of hypoglycemia. There is also the danger of the blood glucose level becoming too high when normal levels of medications are not taken. This can lead to diabetic ketoacidosis (DKA), a condition requiring hospital admission.*

Therefore, you should pay attention to what you eat and try to avoid fasting as much as you can. *Sicknesses have medical cures and you don't have to starve yourself to death for that. And if you are a religious person in search for divine communication or Nirvana, well…maybe your faith is stronger than your health."*

Rebuttal: There is no danger of developing hypoglycemia from fasting. Hypoglycemia is a condition of a low level of glucose in the blood (low blood glucose or "blood sugar"). The endocrine system plays a critical role in glucose metabolism. Two hormones, glucagon and insulin, serve homeostatic roles in maintaining critical levels of glucose in the body for efficient use by body cells. There's actually a cascade of physiological activity aimed at efficient glucose use. Fasting has been used clinically with positive results ending in complete resolution of hypoglycemia.

Dr. Joel Fuhrman, M.D. cites a case of hypoglycemia,

"Samantha, a woman in her early thirties, had such severe hypoglycemic symptoms that she was forced to quit her job. She had seen multiple physicians and had undergone numerous tests. Her fasting glucose level ranged from the forties to 70. She eventually became so weak that she was admitted to the hospital for further evaluation."

"During her evaluation, her doctors could find nothing seriously wrong with her except for unexplained hypoglycemic symptoms. Though still weak she could barely walk, Samantha was discharged from the hospital with instructions to remain on a high-protein diet."

"When Samantha first came to see me she was eating eggs, beef, turkey, ham, and cheese every two hours all day and most of the night. She accompanied each meal with a glass of milk. She could not walk for even two blocks. She was physically disabled, forced to quit her job, and too debilitated to seek any other line of work".

"At the start, I maintained Samantha's eating schedule of every two hours but substituted plant protein for animal protein. Gradually, over the next eight weeks, we eliminated all animal protein. Instead, Samantha ate tofu, beans, lentils, chick peas, lima beans, and pumpkin and sunflower seeds, and increased her intake of green vegetables."

"Over the next few months we made gradual dietary adjustments so that her symptoms would not worsen. Her illness was so severe that I thought she would need to undergo a prolonged fast to completely recover. I was wrong. She made steady progress. The severe incapacitating symptoms slowly resolved, and she soon reported that she had a good energy level. She was able to walk 30 blocks without a problem and has had no further symptoms. She is now back to work, living a normal life."

This case study shows the extraordinary ability of the body to heal when the health-seeker follows a proper diet based upon the biological mandate of the body. Animal proteins (especially cooked proteins) devastate the human body from the inside outwards. Sugar spilling over into the blood and remaining there indicates serious cellular insufficiency to meet the metabolic needs of the body because of long-standing dietary abuse and medical ignorance and mismanagement.

Length of the Fast: Dr. Shelton says, *"In general it may be safely advised that if a fast is undertaken it should be done with satisfactory results as the end in view and stay with it until satisfactory results are forthcoming."*

Fasting should not be entered upon if the health-seeker is frightened of the fast or thinks starvation is an imminent threat. The prejudices against proper fasting are long-standing. It is critical to seek competent guidance from those who are qualified to conduct this method. Giving the body a fair chance to heal and rejuvenate is vital. As long as the body's food reserves are adequate to sustain the inner functioning of cells and organs there is very little threat of starvation. The human body gives the determination of when the fast is nearing its end. Scientists who have witnessed and documented fasters report nothing but beneficial results.

Dr. Shelton documents, *"The usual indications for breaking the fast (these help to determine the dividing line between fasting and starving), are as follow:*
__Hunger__ invariably returns.
The __Breath__, which during all or most of the fast has been offensive, becomes sweet and clean.
The __Tongue__ becomes clean. The thick coating which remained on it throughout most of the fast vanishes.
The __Temperature__, which may have been sub-normal or above normal, returns exactly to normal, where it remains.
The __Pulse__ becomes normal in time and rhythm.
The __Skin__ reactions and other reactions become normal.
The __Bad Taste__ in the mouth ceases.
__Salivary Secretion__ becomes normal.
The __Eyes__ become bright and eye sight improves.
The __Excreta__ loses its odor. The __Urine__ becomes light.

Return of hunger and general physiological re-juvenescence[13] are the best indications that the fast is nearing its end.

Breaking the Fast: Breaking the fast is equally critical as deciding to begin the fast. Overeating after fasting is common among fasters and can be very dangerous. It is important to understand that the stomach has decreased in size and that the food eaten should not threaten the integrity of its structure. It is advised that the foods consumed be efficiently digested and absorbed for optimal use by the body. My recommendations are to use whole foods such as oranges, grapes, watermelon, peaches, and other succulent "juicy" fruits as mono-meals for the first week or so. While it may not always be advisable to fast to completion it is important for the faster to understand that fasting should be carried out long enough to realize the desired results. The body needs to be nourished. Plant foods are superior to animal foods and uncooked foods are superior to cooked foods. Therefore, it behooves the health-seeker to secure those foods which will provide the essential nutrients needed for proper nourishment of body cells.

SUPPLEMENTARY TEXT MATERIAL

The Kidney: Master Organ of Waste Removal, Water Balance, and Salt Balance

Excessive Protein in the Diet Leads to Kidney Failure & Loss

---

[13] Rejuvenescence: is renewal of youth or vitality; in this sense rejuvenescence refers to the on-going process of regeneration on the part of the body to prevent old age and premature death.

The human kidney is exquisitely suited to meet the need of waste removal from the bloodstream and ultimate removal metabolic by-products of metabolism from body. The kidneys are marvels at processing body fluids and filtering out the waste products of metabolism. There are more than a million nephrons[14] packed into each human kidney.

In an adult human, 180 L or more of blood fluid—enough to fill a bathtub—pass through the 2 million nephrons in the two kidneys each day.

The health and optimal functioning of the kidneys depends on the overall wellness of the human body. Chronic Kidney Disease (CKD) is defined either kidney damage or a progressive loss in renal function over a period of months to years. The kidney receives a profuse blood supply. As a consequence, the kidney helps regulate blood pressure, stimulate production of red blood cells, production of hormones such as calcitriol and erythropoietin, and waste removal.

Under the subtitle **Kidney Diseases**[15] in the nation's top selling medical physiology textbook it is stated, *"Diseases of the kidneys are among the most important causes of death and disability in many countries throughout the world. For example, in 2009, more than 26 million adults in the United States were estimated to have chronic kidney disease, and many more millions of people have acute renal failure or less severe forms of kidney dysfunction."*

The devastation of an unwholesome animal-based diet leaves practically **EVERY** body system within the human body in a crippled state. There is raging debate and conflicting research regarding dietary protein and the progression of renal disease. It has been physiologically established that the human kidney is responsible for excreting the products of protein

---

[14] Nephron: The functional unity of the kidney. The nephron is amazingly efficient at removing wastes from the blood circulation while leaving constituents that are critically needed by the body, such as glucose.

[15] **GUYTON AND HALL** Textbook of Medical Physiology 12th Edition

metabolism. Excessive consumption of protein, especially from animal sources, puts a tremendous strain upon the kidney.

The link between high-protein consumption and severe bone-loss (osteoporosis) has also shown a concomitant increase in calcium removal from the body. Obesity is another risk-factor illustrating the link between high-protein ingestion and the artery-clogging fat that is intimately associated with animal-based diets. Heavy animal food consumption places a heavy strain on a hormonal system known as the **"renin-angiotensin system."** Because animal-based diets are severely *water-deficient* there is a constant condition of thirst that is created which forces the consumer into abnormal indulgence of drinking water and other fluids. However, there are many hormones at play which regulate electrolyte *(substances that has the ability to conduct an electric charge + - in solution)* homeostasis. A hormone secreted by the heart called **"Atrial Natriuretic Peptide (ANP)"** is released when blood pressure rises (excessive sodium consumption) which has an opposite effect to the renin-angiotensin system. Atrial natriuretic peptide decreases blood pressure by increasing sodium ($Na+$) and water to flow out of the kidney (*natriuretic* = producing salty urine). Diet plays such a critical role in the health of the kidney. Superior nutrition means *high-level* kidney functioning. One food and **ONLY** one food allow the kidneys to perform their critical role in human physiology unabated: **PLANT FOOD!**

Trick Trition: Lies, Lies, & More Lies...
Chapter 4

This chapter lays the framework for critical analysis of popular claims made for particular foods held up to the public as being critical for the health and well-being of society. I reserve the right to coin or employ a descriptive word or term which exemplifies my criticism made against such claims.

Tricktrition refers to the fraudulent, manipulative, and outright deceptive nutritional information and pseudo-foods flooding the marketplace and landing into the minds of health-seekers with devastating results. We will review and examine some of the most popular claims made for these products.

Pseudo-foods, human-generated nutritional supplements (vitamin, mineral, and herbal), including outright poisons are sold to health-seekers with the promise of increased energy, incredible athletic performance, outstanding intellectual alertness, and overall well-being if consumed on a daily basis. It is scientific certainty that natural law governs the underpinnings of organic and inorganic existence. This means that the nutritional basis of life is governed by an orderly immutable set of principles which dictates the direction in which human wellness should proceed.

Prominent Natural Hygienist and great scientific thinker Herbert M. Shelton wrote a 7-volume series of books known as *"The Hygienic System"* in which he laid down the true nature of disease and the basis in which human wellness is maintained by following a set of living practices in which the laws of nature dictate if health-seekers are to live in superior health. Volume I of this series entitled, *"Orthobionomics"* a term Dr. Shelton coined to reflect the idea that superior health and impaired health are one and the same and, are **NOT** separate entities.

Writing of *"The Laws of Life"* Chapter VI of Orthobionomics Dr. Shelton states,

"The life forces in their operations work, as do all other forces, according to well defined **laws** *or* **uniformities***. Laws have no validity except as expressions of the forces back of them. The uniformities of nature are not mere haphazard coincidences but intrinsically necessary*

conditions. They are based on the nature of things and constitute an intrinsic and necessary part of the world-order, or, rather, of the universal order."

"The uniformities of nature are eternal. They are uncreated and uncreatable. Natural laws are inherent in creation. Man is constituted upon and in perfect harmony with these laws. There is an inseparable and orderly relationship between the laws of nature and the highest welfare of man."

"No one accustomed to observing the exact order and harmony that prevail about him will question that his own body is constituted upon precise and fixed principles and that the vital machinery is controlled by express law."

This statement exemplifies extraordinary internal bodily wisdom. Chemists and scientists "creating" so-called nutritional supplements in a chemical laboratory, packaging them in colorful bottles, defrauding the public out of their hard earned money, causing sickness, disease, premature death and, spewing claims to the public that they'll witness increased body energy and overall well-being is criminal to the nth degree. This *"health-capitalism"* at its best and everyone want a piece of this financial pie.

Is it possible for *"nutritional"* supplements to transmit energy to the body? What about wheatgrass? *"Five-hour"* drinks? There are an endless list of such products and claims on the market which leaves the disillusioned health-seeker experimenting with an endless array of products to the cost of their health and well-being. To explain the appearance of why action occurs when various substances (poisons) are introduced within the human body Dr. Robert Walter another prominent hygienist formulated a set of laws to explain this "action." Let's take a brief look at a few of these laws:

1. **Life's Great Law**: *"Every particle of living matter in the organized body is endowed with an instinct of self-preservation, sustained by a force inherent in the organism, usually called vital force or life, the success of whose work is directly proportioned to the amount of the force and inversely to the degree of its activity."*

2. **The Law of Action**: *"Whenever action occurs in the living organism, as the result of extraneous influences, the action must be ascribed to the living thing, which has the power of action and not to the dead, whose leading characteristic is inertia."*

3. **The Law of Power**: *"The power employed, and consequently expended, in any vital or medicinal action is vital power, that is, power from within and not from without."*

4. **The Law of Dual Effect**: *"The secondary effect upon the living organism of any act, habit, indulgence, or agent is the exact opposite and equal of the primary effect."*

Let's revisit nutritional supplements and the promise of *"increased energy."* First and foremost, when supplements are consumed, there's a very important digestive step completely eliminated: *salivary digestion.* Remember the *cephalic-phase* of digestion? This is critical because neural involvement in preparing the body to handle foodstuffs is very important in how the body efficient handle nutrients. Those who sell supplements for their livelihood perpetuate the outright lie that nutritional supplements increase energy levels.

Let's apply the *"Law of Duel Effect"* to explain this apparent increase of energy health-seekers witness when consuming so-called nutritional and/or herbal supplements.

Dr. Shelton explains, *"Work or exercise arouses vital activity, thus giving an appearance of increased vigor as the first effect. The secondary effect is tiredness, decreased vigor, fatigue, and exhaustion. Rest and sleep on the contrary, produce as their first effect, weakness and languor, but no one doubts their recuperative value. Rest and sleep are the only means whereby recuperation and reinvigoration may be secured. But these are their secondary and lasting effects."*

Consumers of supplements (nutritional & herbal), wheat grass, 5-hour drinks, coffee, and other lesser known pernicious products are promised increased energy and, indeed, they most certainly witness *"increased energy."* This energy that is "felt" leaves the consumer feeling energized, rejuvenated, and refreshed. But, alas, this is the first and temporary effect while the organism marshals its internal resources to expel and eliminate the unwanted, toxic cocktail of these products. But, the secondary and lasting effect is that of weakness, nervousness, psychological, physiological, and emotional drain. Manipulating the human organism with poisons to secure a desired response is an all-time favorite of scientists and those pandering obnoxious products for financial gain.

Shelton explains,

"Self-preservation is the primary or controlling expression of life and, normally, is subordinate to no other law except, at times, to the instinct of race preservation, in which case the individual often sacrifices himself (or herself) for the protection of the young or the flock. Primarily, life seeks to preserve itself and to maintain vital integrity. All functions of life have reference to this effort at self-preservation either of the individual or the race. Nature aims at wholeness. This is as much true of the single cell as of the complex organism."

Dr. Shelton gives a clear and concise explanation why the power of recuperation resides from within the living organism and **NOT** from without saying,

"Power is felt only in its expenditure, never when it is passive. One therefore, feels stronger while he is growing weaker, and feels weaker when he is actually growing stronger, through recuperation of power. The man who has had a drink of alcohol is led to believe that he is strengthened by it, while, in reality, the alcohol has only occasioned the expenditure of the power he possesses. In this way strychnine may "strengthen" the heart until it exhausts this wonderful organ. A cold plunge or a short hot bath produces a general feeling of strength and well-being by occasioning the expenditure of power which they do not and cannot give."

"The thing which seems to give strength is the thing which is taking it away, the thing which appears to be curing the patient is the thing that is hastening his death, the very agents which seem to be "supporting" life are the very things that are undermining the foundations of life."
"Following the period of apparent increase in vigor (stimulation) there comes a period during which there is a feeling of lessened vigor (depression). There are two effects following the use of every force or agent."

The profiteers of the supplementation business wholly and totally disregard the inherent wisdom of physiology. Nature hands humanity foods that are packed with life-sustaining substances in correct proportions for optimal utilization of organismal growth and development. Soil-eating and grass-grazing by humans to obtain "esoteric nutrients" or to find the 'elixir or life' is beyond the height of absurdity. The complex interactions of the various nutrients within the human organism dictate consumption of foods of our biological heritage.

In the next chapter we will explore and identify the specific foods that are considered the best and most optimal to include in the human diet.

We will close this chapter with a comprehensive definition of nutrition by prominent Natural Hygienist Dr. Herbert M. Shelton,

"Nutrition does not mean food only. Nutrition is the sum of all the processes that supply, develop and sustain an organism's faculties and functions at the optimal level of existence. In short, nutrition is the total of all that supplies life's needs. It embraces all requirements for perfect health and supplying these requirements constitutes nutrition."

"Perfect nutrition is dependent on perfect organs, perfect functions and normal health. Each is dependent upon and grows out of the other. All processes and functions are interdependent and interact harmoniously for mutual well-being. They cannot be taken apart and categorized. Every aspect of life is but a part of a unified whole.
This idea of interdependence and interaction leads to the principle that the appropriate way to recover and develop strength and vigor is through the activities and processes that give rise to growth. We recover arid develop strength and vigor in the same way that we keep well, in the same way that a babe grows into vigor and adulthood. The powers and forces that brought us into being, that sustain us in existence, that cause us to grow through all the phases of life to manhood and womanhood, are sufficient to restore us if health becomes impaired."

Superior Nutrition: Life Subject to Law
Chapter 5

What has been said in previous chapters give credence to the fact that the human body is not haphazardly assembled in a disorderly fashion but, instead is governed under strict immutable law. Life means nutrition and nutrition means life.

So, how should we begin our daily dietary regimen? When should we eat? More importantly, what exactly should we eat?

My confirmed recommendation is **DO NOT** follow the *"breakfast, lunch, and dinner scheme."*

- **1st Law**: *Eat ONLY when you are hungry.*

  This first law is critical. Overeating has and continues the devastate the lives of countless men, women, and children. Eating when we are truly hungry allows the mind and body to prepare for the incoming meal and efficiently handle that meal for optimal digestion and absorption.

- **2nd Law**: *Never eat under emotional distress.*

  Extreme emotionalisms such as anger, fear, hate, and any other forms of emotional distress severely (if not completely) suspend the digestion of food. When the digestion of food is delayed in the gastrointestinal system decomposition and/or putrefaction occurs which will eventually put the organism into an eliminative crisis.[16] Under such distress it is critical for the health-seeker to allow complete mental and physiological rest (fasting) until the powers of assimilation (digestion) are restored.

- **3rd Law**: *Consume ONLY pure water.*

  It is critical that the health-seeker understand the benefits of consuming pure water. Distilled water is the purest water. The quality of body tissue and their performance are intimately linked to the quality and quantity of water you drink. Distilled water is FREE from chemical impurities such as vitamins and minerals, pollutants, and other impurities found in so-called 'health" waters sold on the market. The distillation process removes chlorine, nitrites, nitrates, fluorides, ammonia, aluminum, arsenic, copper, iron, mercury, radium, asbestos, so-called viruses, bacteria, herbicides, and pesticides. ONLY DRINK WHEN THIRSTY!

- **4th Law**: *Sunshine.*

---

[16] Eliminative Crisis: Extraordinary effort on the part of the organism to eliminate or rid itself of the generated pinned-up metabolic waste products of metabolism.

Sunshine is a critical element of human nutrition and wellness. Sunbathing on both the front & back side of the body enhances vitamin and calcium metabolism which is necessary for proper bone formation. Secure the beneficial rays of the sunlight at least 20-30 minutes daily, or 2-3 hours per week. Before 10am or after 4pm during the hot summer months, anytime during the cold winter months.

These are only a few of the laws or principles which guides critical development of the human body. We will now list a few other requisites of life which must be observed if we are to attain or reached the pinnacle of our health potential.

- **Fresh Air**
- **Comfortable Body Temperature**
- **Internal & External Cleanliness-** also includes fasting.
- **Rest & Relaxation-** physical, physiological, and sensory rest. (Fasting)
- **Sleep**
- **Proper Food: Consuming Foods of our Biological Adaptation**
- **Exercise-** at least 3-4 times per week.
- **Play & Recreation**
- **Mental Poise**
- **Security of Life and Its Means**
- **Creative Work**
- **Self-Mastery**
- **Peer Interaction-** importance of positive involvement with others.
- **Expression of Reproductive Instinct**
- **Love, Appreciation, Positive Self-Esteem**
- **Appreciation of Beauty**
- **Inspiration & Motivation**

Questions from Health Seekers

Question: *With so much information on health today how can I know which diet is right for me?*

Answer: As scientists and professionals of nutritional science it is critical that we seek an understanding of not only how the body functions but the precise nutritional needs of the body based upon biological evidence. Comparative anatomy and physiology provides evidence of the proper foods for humans. Nature decrees that we adhere to a plant-based diet for optimal wellness. The idea that humans should consume any and everything that crawls upon and underneath the surface of the earth as promoted by the meat-packing and dairy industries has caused countless premature deaths.

Question: *The diet that you recommend and promote would be very difficult for most people to adhere to. How can we follow such a diet without getting bored?*

Answer: According to Wikipedia, the free encyclopedia, **Boredom** is *"an emotional state experienced when an individual is left without anything in particular to do, and not interested in their surroundings."* This definition **DOES NOT** describe an individual who is "truly hungry." Nature hands us an enormous variety of delectable and colorful foods for our enjoyment and satisfaction. Consuming foods in consonance with our biological requirements satisfies many other requisites of life such as the appreciation of beauty, olfactory (smell of delectable flavors) and sensory fulfillment. We cannot appreciate these facets with the destructiveness that consuming animal foods afford.

Question: *Why do you recommend an all raw plant-based diet? I was under the impression that food should be cooked to kill germs, bacteria, and viruses?*

Answer: Nutritionally raw or uncooked foods are superior to cooked foods in every respect. As explained in the body of the book the human body needs various nutrients to conduct important physiological activities for its very survival. Consuming cooked foods handicaps the body on many levels. Even the structure of the teeth shows weakness from the aftermath of eating predominantly of cooked foods as the primary method of consumption. Under most circumstances cooking renders food unfit for human consumption.

The idea that germs and other microorganisms should be killed to render food safe for consumption is a medical delusion. This claim is also the basis for food irradiation. Microorganisms serve a very critical symbiotic role to the host organism such as host defense and enteric[17] generation of certain vitamins.

Question: *Health professionals say that following a complete plant-based diet is nutritionally inadequate and should be supplemented with a multi-vitamin supplement. Do you recommend nutritional supplements as part of a healthy diet?*

Answer: The supplementation business is a multi-billion dollar racket. While those who consume supplements continue to suffer with symptoms of ill health the profits from the sale of this deadly exploitation continues to get dumped into the coffers of those who stand to profit handsomely from an ill-informed gullible public. So-called *"nutritional supplements"* are non-usable and present a serious eliminative burden on the body must deal with or store for future elimination. The biological scheme of food consumption and elimination is utterly and completely ignored by the panderers of supplements. Eating soil as a means nutritional acquisition is utter nonsense. Supplements should NEVER be part of a healthy diet or lifestyle.

---

[17] Enteric: is a term usually used in association with the intestine. Enteritis refers to inflammation of the intestines.

Question: *What about growing children wouldn't they need animal foods for extra protein?*

Answer: Children indeed need nutrients for their rapid growth and development. Animal foods are a major factor in the epidemic of chronic illness in this country. Children are physically very active and this activity is powered by consumption of carbohydrate-rich foods such as fruits, vegetables, and nuts. Each stage of human development from infancy to adulthood determines the amount of protein needed for optimal wellness. Protein is need most during infancy because of rapid growth and development and the amount decreases with growth and maturity. Eating animal protein over exceeds human enzyme digestion.

Question: *You spoke briefly about fasting is really any value to fasting?*

Answer: In the animal kingdom fasting is employed for various reasons. Animals may fast during their mating season, during food scarcity, injury, and/or illness. Likewise, humans have physiological and psychological mechanisms that allow for this life-saving process. Fasting should <u>NEVER</u> be looked upon as a curative measure for illness. Fasting affords the body a definite period of complete rest. During this period of rest the body actively accelerates it's eliminative for the expulsion of waste products, poisons from drugs and other deadly chemicals, and other debris that cripples the integrity of the organism. I refer health-seekers to works of the late Dr. Herbert M. Shelton for further in-depth research on fasting and on the tremendous benefits of Natural Hygiene.

Food-Combining Rules for MAXIMUM Health Results!

Following the rules herein are pertinent to the success of achieving high-level health and especially for the maximum digestion of foods eaten. With our current understanding of digestive chemistry we can intelligently lay the foundation for a rational approach for nourishing the human body. Observation of these food-combining rules is the cornerstone of success to your road to success.

Rule# 1: Melons (Eat Alone or Let Alone)

Why should we eat melons alone on an empty stomach?

Dr. Vivian Vetrano states:
"Melons are best taken alone because the sugar and other nutriments are in a less stable form than the nutriments of other fruits. Orange juice may be kept in the refrigerator for an hour with little change in flavor, but if you refrigerate watermelon juice for only ten minutes, its flavor and color and composition change. It decomposes much more quickly than other fruits. Consequently, if it is held in the stomach awaiting the digestion of other foods, it will decompose (ferment) and cause a great deal of gastric distress. Eating watermelon with nuts can readily be troublesome. One should not take watermelon with other more concentrated fruits. The more concentrated the food is, the longer it takes to propel it from the stomach, and if the melon is held in the stomach mixed with the other fruit, then it also will be held in the stomach for a longer period of time. Watermelon must be evacuated from the stomach as rapidly as it would be if eaten alone. If eaten with other foods that slow its evacuation time from the stomach then it will ferment in the stomach and cause trouble."

The body handles fruit with such ease and efficiency that it is my confirmed recommendation that melons are eaten alone and fruits in general are eaten on an empty stomach. This approach prevents bacterial fermentation of fruit sugars and the consequent digestive troubles and other disturbances that are the result of combining fruits with other foods.

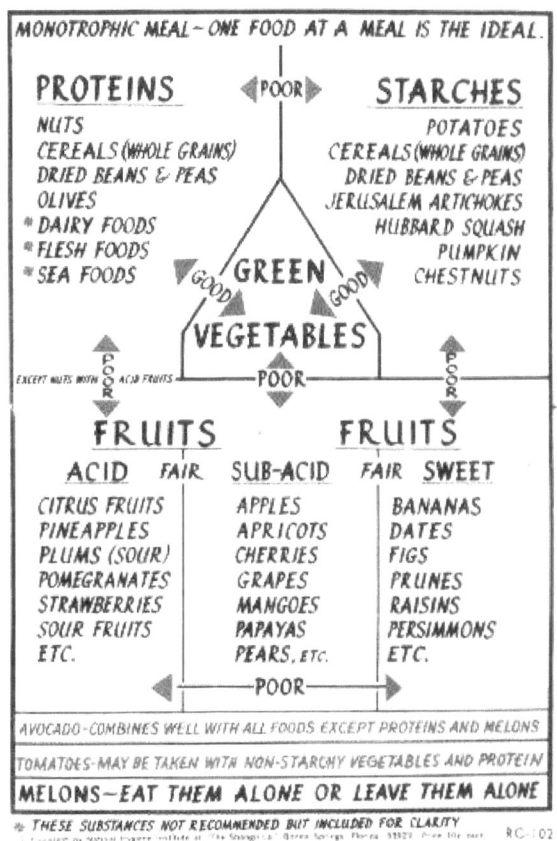

CORRECT FOOD COMBINING

MONOTROPHIC MEAL – ONE FOOD AT A MEAL IS THE IDEAL.

PROTEINS	◀POOR▶	STARCHES
NUTS		POTATOES
CEREALS (WHOLE GRAINS)		CEREALS (WHOLE GRAINS)
DRIED BEANS & PEAS		DRIED BEANS & PEAS
OLIVES		JERUSALEM ARTICHOKES
* DAIRY FOODS		HUBBARD SQUASH
* FLESH FOODS		PUMPKIN
* SEA FOODS	GOOD▼ GREEN ▲GOOD	CHESTNUTS

GREEN VEGETABLES

EXCEPT NUTS WITH ACID FRUITS ——— POOR ———

FRUITS   FRUITS

ACID   FAIR   SUB-ACID   FAIR   SWEET

ACID	SUB-ACID	SWEET
CITRUS FRUITS	APPLES	BANANAS
PINEAPPLES	APRICOTS	DATES
PLUMS (SOUR)	CHERRIES	FIGS
POMEGRANATES	GRAPES	PRUNES
STRAWBERRIES	MANGOES	RAISINS
SOUR FRUITS	PAPAYAS	PERSIMMONS
ETC.	PEARS, ETC.	ETC.

◀———— POOR ————▶

AVOCADO - COMBINES WELL WITH ALL FOODS EXCEPT PROTEINS AND MELONS

TOMATOES - MAY BE TAKEN WITH NON-STARCHY VEGETABLES AND PROTEIN

MELONS—EAT THEM ALONE OR LEAVE THEM ALONE

* THESE SUBSTANCES NOT RECOMMENDED BUT INCLUDED FOR CLARITY

RC-102

Proper food-combining provides the health-seeker with a sound physiological method to insure efficient digestion of foods eaten. Carefully study the food-combining charts and put the principles of correct biological eating in your everyday dietary regimen.

1. *Never eat carbohydrate foods at the same meal.*

2. *Never eat a concentrated protein and a concentrated carbohydrate at the same meal.*

3. *Never consume two concentrated proteins at the same meal.*

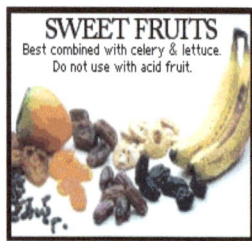

SWEET FRUITS
Best combined with celery & lettuce.
Do not use with acid fruit.

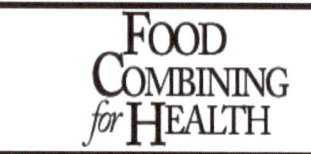

FOOD COMBINING for HEALTH

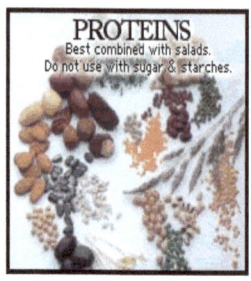

PROTEINS
Best combined with salads.
Do not use with sugar & starches.

SUB-ACID FRUITS
Combined with acid or sweet fruits, but not both. Good with lettuce or celery.

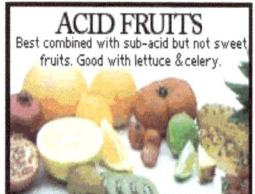

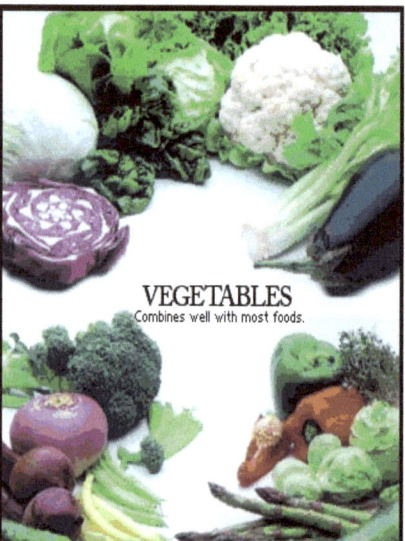

VEGETABLES
Combines well with most foods.

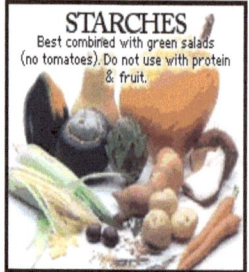

STARCHES
Best combined with green salads
(no tomatoes). Do not use with protein
& fruit.

ACID FRUITS
Best combined with sub-acid but not sweet
fruits. Good with lettuce & celery.

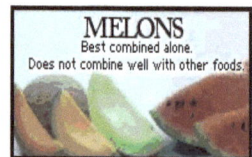

MELONS
Best combined alone.
Does not combine well with other foods.

4. *Do not consume fats with proteins.*

5. *Use fats sparingly.*

6. *Do not eat acid fruits with proteins.*

7. *Do not combine sweet fruits that require a long digestive time- foods such as proteins, starches, and acid fruits.*

8. *Eat but one concentrated starch at a meal.*

9. *Acid fruits may be used with sub-acid fruits.*

10. *Sub-acid fruits may be used with sweet fruits.*

11. *Do not combine fruit with any vegetables except lettuce and celery.*

12. Salads combine very well with proteins or starches.

13. Do not consume melons with any other foods. (Eat melons alone)

14. Alfalfa sprouts may be combined as a green vegetable.

15. Milk is best consumed alone on an empty stomach.

Food-combining is based upon sound physiological digestive chemistry. Whether the health-seeker is following a plant-based diet or a mixed diet of plant and animal foods the principles of food-combining should be utilized to maintain the integrity of the digestive system and overall health of the consumer. Meal-planning should be simple and easy to craft. Follow the instructions given within the pages of this book and you will begin to witness high-level superlative health, increased energy, and total well-being from the inside/out.

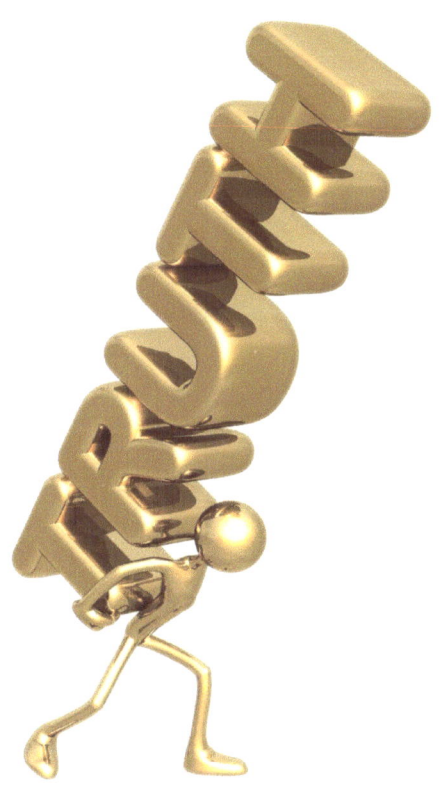

Food Combinations & Choices

Color-coding: **Green** means recommended, **red** means discouraged. Shades between indicate points on sliding scale.

POOR

PROTEINS[2,4]

Avocado	*Turkey, Fish,*
Coconut	*Beef, Venison,*
Dairy[3] *(Cheese,*	*Pork, etc)*
Cottage Cheese,	**Nuts**
Ice Cream, Milk,	**Olives**
Yogurt.	**Seeds**
Eggs	**Soybeans**
Meat *(Chicken,*	

FATS & OILS

Avocado Oil	Olive Oil
Butter	Safflower Oil
Canola Oil	Green Tea
Coconut Oil	Seed Oil
Corn Oil	Soy Oil
Cream	Sesame Oil
Lard	
Nut Oils	

CARBOHYDRATES[2]

Beans	Pumpkin
Bread	Split Peas
Brown Rice	Squash *(acorn,*
Cereals	*banana, hub-*
Grains[6]	*bard)*
Lentils	Wheat[8]
Pastas	White Rice
Potatoes	

POOR   **GOOD**

EXCELLENT

NON-STARCHY VEGETABLES

Asparagus	Eggplant	Radishes
Beet Greens	Endive	Scallions
Broccoli	Escarole	Spinach
Brussels Sprouts	Garlic	Sprouts
Cabbage	Green Beans	Summer Squash
Celery	Kale	Sweet Pepper
Chard	Kohlrabi	Swiss Chard
Chicory	Leeks	Tomatoes
Collards	Lettuce	Turnips
Cucumber	Onions	Watercress
Dandelion	Parsley	Zucchini

GOOD   **EXCELLENT**   **EXCELLENT**   **GOOD**

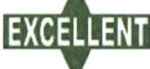

EXCELLENT

MILDLY-STARCHY VEGETABLES

Artichokes	Carrots	Corn
Beets	Cauliflower	Peas

GOOD   **GOOD**

ACID FRUIT

Blackberry	Plum (sour)
Grapefruit	Pomegranate
Lemon/Lime	Raspberry
Orange	Sour Apple
Pineapple	Strawberry

SUB-ACID FRUIT

Apple	Mango
Apricot	Peach
Blueberry	Pear
Cherry	Plum
Kiwi	(sweet)

SWEET FRUIT

Bananas	Papaya
Dates	Persimmon
Currants	Prunes
Figs	Raisins
Grapes	

MELON

Cantaloupe	Watermelon
Casaba	
Crenshaw	
Honeydew	
Persian	

FRUITS are best when eaten **alone**, as a meal, when the stomach is empty of other foods, such as for breakfast. Each fruit group should be eaten separately from other fruit groups, especially melons and sweet fruits.

NOTES

1. ALSO REFER TO ALKALINE/ACID FOODS CHART
2. Carbohydrates and Proteins should never be eaten together, or during the same meal period.
3. Milk and other dairy products are discouraged for human consumption *(Exception: mother's breast milk is highly recommended for babies of the same species!)*
4. Concentrated proteins are unnecessary. Use as a condiment, not as main course. In any case, eat **no more than** one each meal.
5. Garlic has been reported to produce adverse side effects, and should be considered for medicinal use only.
6. **Good** when sprouted to vegetable state before consumption.
7. *"All things in moderation, including moderation."* Socrates
8. This information may be copied and distributed freely.

Notes/ Questions

TOUCHED BY HEALTH®

Services offered: (Free Initial 20/min. Consultation)

- **Personal Consultations** (Basic charge is $2.00/min.)
  Minimum consultation fee is $20.00 for 10/min. or under. Hourly consultation fee is

- **Personalized Dietary Plans/ Exercise Programs**
  There is a $100.00 fee for weekly dietary/exercise programs and/or $375 for monthly dietary/exercise programs (save $25 for monthly program). The fees quoted are separate from the consultation fees.

  Please Note: Dietary/Exercise programs can be purchased separately.

- **Health Seminars/ Speaking Engagements**
  Health seminars and/or speaking engagements are based on a sliding scale between $200- $2,500 based upon length of time, distance of travel, urgency, and preparation of program.

- **Family Plan**
  Family consultations are available with a 5% discount off regular fee.

  All fees are subject to a sliding scale and are therefore subject to change. For further information about other services offered by **Touched by Health®** please contact instructor:

  Curtis Roberson
  (216)804.0580
  sheltonianthinker@yahoo.com

  Method of payment: At this time cash and/or money order will be accepted as the method of payment.

Touched by Health®
INSTITUTE OF NUTRITIONAL SCIENCE

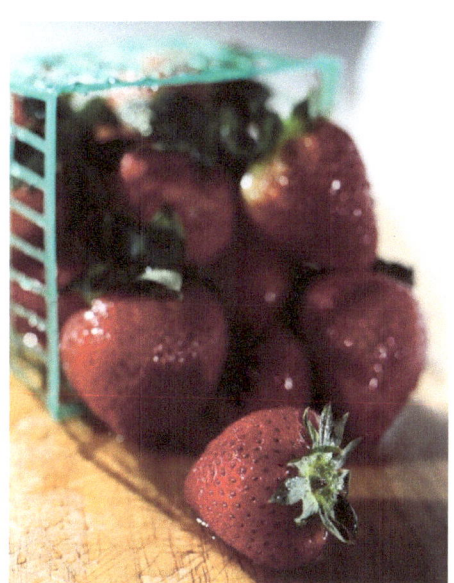

25% off Discount Coupon

This coupon is valid for the first initial visit which includes the interview, evaluation, and 20 min. consultation.

Offered exclusively by:
Touched by Health®
Educational/Research Institute of Nutritional Science
Curtis Roberson
(216)804.0580
sheltonianthinker@yahoo.com

References and Suggested Readings

1. T. Colin Campbell PhD with Thomas M. Campbell II. <u>The China Study</u>. *"Startling Implications for Diet, Weight Loss and Long-Term Health."* (2004)

2. Joel Fuhrman, M.D. <u>Fasting and Eating for Health</u>. *"A Medical Doctor's Program for Conquering Disease."* (1995).

3. Frank A. Oski, M.D. **Don't** <u>Drink Your Milk</u>. *"New Frightening Medical Facts about the World's Most Overrated Nutrient."* TEACH Services, Inc. (1996).

4. Herbert M. Shelton. *<u>Exercise</u>*. Natural Hygiene Press, Inc. (1971).

5. Herbert M. Shelton. *<u>The Science and Fine Art of Fasting.</u>* American Natural Hygiene Society, Incorporated, 1993.

6. Herbert M. Shelton. *<u>Fasting Can Save Your Life</u>*. Natural Hygiene Press, Inc. (1964).

7. Herbert M. Shelton. *<u>Food Combining Made Easy</u>*. Willow Publishing, Inc. (1997).

8. William Esser. *<u>Dictionary of Natural Foods</u>*. Natural Hygiene Press. (1983).

9. Groff, James L., Sareen S. Gropper, and Sara M. Hunt. *<u>Advanced Nutrition and Human Metabolism</u>*. West Publishing Company. (1995).

10. Koeppen, M. Bruce, and Bruce A. Stanton. *<u>Berne & Levy Physiology 6th Ed</u>*. Mosby, Inc. (2008).

11. Hall, E. John. *<u>Guyton and Hall Textbook of Medical Physiology</u>*. Elsevier, Inc. (2011).

12. Fry, TC. *<u>The Great Power Within You</u>*. Life Science: "Lesson Number One."

VEGAN NUTRITION: The Raw Truth

This is the first book of its kind to provide health-seekers with an understandable explanation of how the body actually function giving the reader a critical backdrop to the nutritional soundness of plant-based nutrition. The reader is taken step-by-step through an exciting journey into the body and what actually happens to food when it is eaten. There are many examples of why plant foods are superior to animal foods.